KYOTO SAKURA

Copyright 2017

Printed in The U.S.A.

All right reserved. This Coloring books or any potion thereof many not be reproduced or used in any manner whatsoever without the exoress written permission of the publisher except.

TEST YOUR COLOR

1.

www.ingramcontent.com/pod-product-compliance
Lightning Source LLC
Chambersburg PA
CBHW081213180526
45170CB00006B/2327